MEDICAL POEMS

MEDICAL POEMS

BENEDICT OF MILAN

DALCASSIAN PRESS
Dark Age & Medieval Texts

Translator: Curtin, D.P. (1985-)

ISBN: 979-8-3495-2628-2 (Paperback)
ISBN: 979-8-3495-2627-5 (eBook)
Library of Congress Control Number:

Printed by Ingram Content Group, 1 Ingram Blvd, La Vergne, Tennessee
First Printing 2020, Dalcassian Press, Wilmington, DE

This work is part of a series produced in association with the Scriptorium Project and its community of scholars and translators.
Please visit our website at: www.thescriptoriumproject.com

1

MEDICAL POEMS

CRIPSUS THE DEACON OF MILAN TO MAURUS MANTUENSEM PREFACE TO THE BOOK OF MEDICINE.

Since I have almost raised you, dearest son Maurus, from your very cradle, and enriched you with the bounty of sevenfold eloquence, there is one thing that you have always wished to remain ungrateful for in your flourishing years, which is the skill of medicine, despising it in all respects, saying that you retain no part or communion in the liberal arts; but now, since the enormity of various ailments often dominates you, you are compelled to enhance the same arts with skill, which you were not ashamed to call nefarious and most disgraceful before. Therefore, you demand that I make you a countryman, teaching you the virtues of medicinal herbs, and that I show them individually at certain times, and, according to the various qualities of ailments, I will undoubtedly present the types of cures. I willingly accepted your annual request; and, striving for brevity in this present work, I wish to nourish you with heroic honey, so that I may gradually lead you to the love of the art; lest if I unfold too many things at first, the plurality may cause disgust, and disgust may take away desire. Therefore, what I have deemed most excellent, I have briefly summarized; so that while you prove these things to be true in the clearest work, you may more ardently and diligently pursue the many that remain.

I. ON THE HEAD.

If the head is troubled by countless throbbings,
And is disturbed by a certain encircling weight,
At once strive to crown it with ivy.
Thus also when it is joined with dreadful vinegar.
Myrrh is also united with liquid olive,
And the famous cephalota with savory salt.
However, a part of it shakes if troubled by disease,
The active mole is captured, which digests all oil,
And the head and face will be anointed with the oil of which.

II. ON TOOTHACHE.

But if the many-toothed are shaken by a whirlwind,
The strong symphony is pressed with the thumb of the tooth:
At once all raging pain will depart.
Yet I warn you not to swallow, because the treacherous plague
Seizes the sense when taken, captured like the image of death.
If, however, the insane throat seizes and shakes with cold,
A drink will be a remedy, a healing ointment.

III. ON PHRENZY.

But if an immense pain penetrates the meninges,
And the brain is corrupted by the rampaging malediction of phrenzy,
Pleasant will be the lung taken from the viscera of a deer
Mixed with the head, or the power of drunk coriander,
Or the skin of radish softened with fierce vinegar:
The bitter one is too sharp, but certainly an ancient remedy.

IV. ON THE EYES.

Without a doubt, swift languor corrupts the quick orbs,
And fortune burns troubled in various ways:
For it injures, but the loving one heals with a certain time.
Therefore, at once prepare boiled marrubium,
You tie together betonica, and also the juicy wool:
It quickly removes all evil, restoring the pious light.
If there is a red pain in the eyes stirred by moisture,
Then the powerful verbena will be drunk with a gentle wave.

V. ON THE SPOT IN THE EYE.

If you retain a spot in the eyes while rolling inward,
Look while you go along the red slime through the fields,
Which pouring from the eye, prepare a certain modicum.

VI. ON THE ANGINA OF THE THROAT.

But if the angina has invaded the ample throat,
And has filled it with swollen leaves,
Arsenicon is ground with joined pepper and clay,
Thus placed, it is blown through the rough throat.

VII. ON THE GRAPE OF THE THROAT.

The grape, when ripe, if it does not contain the measure itself,
Drips heavy and putrid drops into the body,
It badly pierces the light of the lungs with filthy wings,
It is dried more quickly from the raging dust.

VIII. ON HEALING THE LUNG.

Often the very force of man shakes the thorax itself,
And it is seen to threaten many with dire death.
If you wish, therefore, to polish the sick thorax with care,
Do not hesitate to consider the various cures of herbs.
Wool soaked in oil, as well as the juice of Greek fenugreek,
These restore the stomach, as does the drink of myrica,

The famous brassica is joined with betonica,
The radish from milk, also the juice of the green one must be given.
And the famous lelisphagus herb is also taken,
Thus the final great remedy of cedar will be given.

IX. ON HEARTACHE.

When insane pain beats against the side of the chest,
And the fibers of the heart are greatly tormented by bitter pain,
Dire streams help when joined with the virtue of coral.
Then the light pipinella is joined by the right of marathrum.
Sizaduar is captured, as well as masculine tanacetum,
Which also calms fever and repels the poisons of the heart.

X. ON THE CURE OF PLEURISY.

But if a great disease has struck the pious side,
And life is troubled by a double peril,
You should strive to hasten the skin of the wolf, and place hot,
You will be able to use the marrow of the deer with the oil of the goat.
At once let them be placed in a pot, and with slow fire,
Pitch is also joined with britia and boiled,
Along with flour and the very wolf, and not without saffron.
Thus let the pious poultice be joined with the bitter disease,
So that rest may be given to the wretched laboring man.
And the famous remedy of Tonantis repels the malady.

XI. ON THE CURE OF THE SPLEEN.

The swollen spleen then troubles a man with a heavy burden,
Cook betonica, and the purified doves as companions,
Which two joined together demand to be united with cephalota,
And rosy oil; thus surely you tie together the soaked.
Short thyme is seized, and lupins are joined,
And often they are given, and the tongue of the deer is also drunk,

By which virtue the face perishes, but is gently wrinkled.
It is born in the stones humble, but it is great for the spleen
And friendly to man, but not suitable for laughter.
As many as there are members of man, so many are the plagues in the body.
But powerful medicine restrains many with its service.
While the liver is corrupted and glides like a scyrosis,
Bitter costus is drunk, and also the great reubarbarus.
Which, when crushed together, repress the swelling with salt.
The lupine fiber is strong, it helps and is good for the suffering,
When the liver suffers on the right, the spleen itself on the left.
Therefore, the care of both is equally joined to both.

XII. ON STOMACH AND INTESTINAL PAINS.

The innermost viscera are shaken in various ways by pain,
And the whole sick person is tormented by threatening languor,
Nor does any hope of life remain, when the very spirit
Seeks the heights, a wanderer departs, leaving behind all good things.
This is said to be twisted, because it torments the heavy viscera,
And again and again it calms, all
Beloved nature is simultaneously corrupted, what the fervent lymph restores.
Thus, sluggish limbs are nourished by its liquor
And all the cold are nourished by the flowing warmth.
Afterwards, the fat of the goose is poured out,
And the combined virtue of Greek fenugreek is revealed.
No less is the very force of the flowing liquid cooked.
Immediately, a fearful clyster is poured into the anus,
By which virtue the wretched may be able to restore the pain
Caused by squibala when there is no healthy remedy,
And it closes the narrow course of the suffering cholera.
The snowy elephant is scraped, and immediately it is drunk,

This potion quickly untwists the twisted.
Puppies are taken as it is said, the pious blind viscera,
Thus, soft little limbs should be applied to tender fibers.
And all pain passes into the viscera of the split.
Pliny records this, we know who spoke the truth.

XIII. ON THE TREATMENT OF DROPSY.

From the scyros spleens, a mortal humor is born,
And it segregates the miserable skin from the miserable viscera,
And such is the force of the disease, that thirst is never satisfied.
Ashes are taken, which the tall ash burns,
From these, the hard barley is broken,
Twice boiled, it is faithfully mixed for the suffering,
Radish is ordered with the best sweet honey,
From whose leaves the epithem is applied to it.
Sulfur is drunk with old hot wine:
No less, from the very ones, apply the epithem to the swollen.
These dissolve scyrosin from the spleens, and also dry the lymphs.

XIV. ON THE WORMS.

If wounds fester with putrid blood,
It is fitting to drink hot goat's milk
And no less does it dissolve the dreadful abscess from the she-ass.
The ashes of the vine are poured out with olive oil:
This drink is worthy of many putrid things through the ages.
But also celery and figs, as well as laurel berries,
Iris, and the great Illyrian centaury rue,
These will be able to wipe away the purulent filth more quickly,
And restore the revived man in joyful days.

XV. ON EAR WORMS.

It is fitting for the heedless to pretend to be cautious,
So that the bodies may not be disturbed by the untrained sense.

When immense sleep has pervaded the limbs of man,
Then it is usual for unworthy animals to penetrate the ears.
Take quickly with onion or vinegar from mice,
And do not delay, thus you will be able to drive away the worm.

XVI. ON DEAFNESS.

But if you suffer from deafness, read the red worms
Of the ancient tree, thus mix them with pure olive oil;
Pour into the ears, return eager health to you.
The fat of the goose is beneficial and that of the black vulture.
The juice of onions helps the ears and provides good,
When the lymph usually penetrates the careless ears.

XVII. ON DYSENTERY.

Often the excessive course of the belly tends to overflow,
Gradually dissolving the tender flesh of many,
Whom the prudent medicine of God knows how to restrain.
Asian gall is helpful, as is the long cherry fruit,
Cheese will be suitable with the sweet gift of honey,
And warm fat from the ruptured goat will benefit
When placed on the belly, a remedy that is well known.
But if by chance it drops a nail from itself,
It signifies that it quickly desires to lose life.

XVIII. ON HARDNESS OF THE BELLY.

If indeed the belly is disturbed by immense weight,
Look at where it grows, hunting for the seed of Pallas;
This virgin is said to be friendly to all and a friend of health;
Immediately and the head, good grace swells in the belly.
Hellebore is taken, crushed, and honey is drunk,
Always this has been useful for this disease, and also with chamomile
Diluted with old wine should be drunk immediately.

The taste of horse milk will also benefit without delay.
Eupator, prasion, and hermodactylus itself,
As it is said in books, are always friends of the belly.

XIX. ON THE BLADDER.

Many things help many because they are contrary to diseases
The disease is overcome by the antidote of the high god.
There is a species of disease and a pest that is hostile to many,
When the burning calculus of the bladder rages madly,
Indeed generating stones with which urine hesitates.
Nor does the suffering man have the power to release kind rains.
The tall ivy will give berries from its lofty summit,
And take its juice with warm wine,
And without delay, the plantain of the acorn will burst, and it itself
Is taken and drunk, and the kind olusatrum.
They carry away saxifrage from the stone and also from celery.
By these votes, you will be supported. And you will ask the Lord.

XX. ON THE FLOW OF URINE.

But if, on the contrary, it has poured out excessive rains,
Immediately restrain the flow from the brain of the hare.
You take old wines, when you perceive the brain itself,
Indeed, it is cheap to drink, but not cheap as a remedy.

XXI. ON NOSE BLEEDING.

It should be said to all when the wave of blood pours out
From the nose of the hemorrhoid, which is a certain hope of health.
Rue will give a drink equally crushed with odor,
The humble from the fields is beneficial when crushed with cumin
Of hypporis, and it stops the blood from flowing from the joined nostril
With the powder of the mushroom which they say is lupine,

You also associate the cheap grasses of mint with the nostrils.

XXII. ON HEMORRHOIDS.

But if the obscene disease has attempted the anus,
Let the powerful maurella, hostile to the mole, be sought,
And also hyosciamus, of which a healthy cure is made
These, when drunk together, already stop the blood
Lead and burnt oil is harmful when joined with moist olive.
By these two together, the wave of blood stands still.

XXIII. ON FIRE.

The fierce fire always rages, burning the viscera,
And it always wanders, releasing a fierce flame beneath the skin
And again leaping, swelling under the image of a fountain.
Let the mind of man always be ready against its internal frauds;
It is pleasing to smear with the herb of chelidonia.
The internal is joined with the snowy white of the egg,
Rue helps and drives away the disease, and also tightens the flame,
If it is joined at the same time with warm and pure olive oil.
Do not think that I speak falsely, when the truth
Itself commands; produce the dung of the sheep with the disease
And that warm, which many report in song.

XXIV. ON CARBON.

The hostile disease thrives when the huge coal rages,
Terrifyingly it destroys the innards when it seizes.
To this, the essence of Jove's beard and likewise benign,
Which is at once an enemy, and also crushed savin
Is drunk with the dung of the shining dove's laws;
If taken, it remains trembling in the body's belly,
Life's salvation is thus promised to the fearful sick.
But if it seems exhausted, it appears to reject the drink,
Believe me, it seems to reveal swift death.

This dreadful seed of ravages is also expelled,
Quintus asserts this with true reasoning, Serenus.
Imprinted cauteries benefit the disease with severity,
Lime also alive is immediately scattered in it.
And when a red scar has been commanded by God,
Then truly, undaunted, compose the timid care,
So that the virulent plague may be able to draw in poisons.
I attest this, you should know to avoid sleep,
Lest the fearsome revived be able to restore vigor.

XXV. ON ARTHRITIC SCIATICA.

If the hip has deprived someone of their step,
And furious moisture has grown through the bones,
Take the polypody which they say is a fern,
To which the crushed black clove is well mixed,
Ductile and pepper, pleasing cinnamon to all.
Thus make the drink; but grant it not without honey.
Learn to seek the book of the elm tree,
To which mix the ruby, then drink joyfully.
Seeing the nettle of the field, do not scorn the greater,
Which, when drunk for a long time, knows to burn the pest.
Hold this certain, firm, and true, my son.

XXVI. ON CURING GOUT.

Many bring forth much, whose writing is healthful,
Who, however, assert that the sluggish gout is without care,
To say if it is possible; if you wish to help the disease,
Begin what I advise; cut the pleasant milk thistles.
Thus the immense pain knows to overcome pain.
The happy ointment gives rest to the steps,
And the powerful myrica, also the living little beard of Jove,
Are equally applied, are bound to the feet, and they themselves
Are continually given as drink to the lame.

Do you wish to now entrust miraculous health to yourself?
Catch the little fish called ruccas by name.
Which, placed on the side, add to the burning coals,
Compose the steps and the certain hot ones of the suffering;
They repress every evil, thus the harsh pest is driven away.

THE WORK OF CRISPUS THE DEACON OF MILAN TO MACRUS THE PREPOSITUS OF MANTUA IS COMPLETE. BUT INDEED THIS CRISPUS IS NEITHER A POET NOR A GOOD VERSIFIER; FOR HE COMPOSED VERSES NOT ACCORDING TO THE LAW OF METERS BUT TO THE SOUND OF HIS OWN EARS, THAT IS, ONLY RHYTHM.

THE END.

2

LATIN TEXT

CRISPI MEDIOLANENSIS DIACONI AD MAURUM MANTUENSEM PRAEPOSITUM IN MEDICINAE LIBELLUM PRAEFATIO.

Quia te, fili charissime Maure, pene ab ipsis cunabulis educavi, et septiformis facundiae liberalitate ditavi, unum tibi deest quod adhuc in annis virentibus constitutus ingratum semper habere voluisti, hoc est gratae peritiam medicinae per omnia parvipendens, nullam in liberalibus disciplinis partem communionemque retinere dixisti; nunc autem quia valetudinum variarum saepius in te dominatur enormitas, cogis ipsam eamdem artium amplificare peritiae, quam prius non erubuisti nefariam et turpissimam nuncupare. Exigis ergo a me ut te ruricolam faciam, herbarum medicinalium virtutes edoceam, ipsasque temporibus certis singillatim ostendam, et, juxta valetudinum multiplices qualitates, species curationum indubitanter exhibeam. Quod tuae annuens voluntati libenter excepi; et, breviloquio in praesenti opusculo studens, heroico te melle pascere cupio, ut paulatim ad artis amorem adducam; ne si plura primitus in os tendendo retexero, pluralitas fastidium faciat, fastidium desiderium tollat. Ergo quod probatissimum habeo succincta supputatione perstrinxi; ut dum ista opere liquidissimo vera esse probaveris, plurima quae restant ardentius atque diligentius assequaris.

I. DE CAPITE.

Si caput innumeris agitatur pulsibus aegrum,
Ac circumflexo turbatur pondere quodam,
Protinus ex hederae studeas redimire corona.
Thus quoque cum diro Libanum copulatur aceto.
Myrrha etiam liquido pariter sociatur olivo,
Et cephalota simul celebris cum sale savina.
Pars tamen ex ipso quatitur si concita morbo,
Talpa vigens capitur, oleum quam concoquat omne,
Et caput et facies linietur unguine de quo.

II. DE DENTIUM DOLORE.

At si multiphagi quatiuntur turbine dentes,
Symphoniaca valens premitur cum pollice denti:
Protinus ex ipso rabidus dolor omnis abibit.
Ne glutias tamen admoneo, quia perfida pestis
Sumpta rapit sensum, capitur quasi mortis imago.
Si vero insanus guttur rapit et quatit algens,
Sister erit potus, unguen medicina salubris.

III. DE PHRENESI.

At dolor immensus penetrat si forte meningas,
Et vitiat cerebrum grassans maledicta phrenesis,
Gratus erit pulmo sumptus de viscere cervi
Compositus cephalo, seu vis epota corandri,
Aut raphani cortex saevo mollitus aceto:
Sumptus acer nimium est, sed certe cura vetusta.

IV. DE OCULIS.

Haud dubium celeres vitiat languor citus orbes,

Et variis turbata modis fortuna perurget:
Laedit enim, sed curat amans cum tempore certo.
Ergo age marrubium statim componito coctum,
Betonicam nectis certus, sucidam quoque lanam:
Omne malum tollit citius, pia lumina reddit.
Si dolor est oculis rubeus quem concitat humor,
Tum verbena potens leni potabitur unda.

V. DE MACULA OCULI.

Si maculam retines oculis, dum volvitur intro,
Conspice dum pergis rubeum per rura limacem,
Quem fundens oculo modium componito certus.

VI. DE ANGINA GUTTURIS.

Si vero angina guttur pervaserit amplum,
Ac foliis tumidis arcens compleverit illud,
Arsenicon teritur juncto pipere boloque,
Sic positum pennae perflatur gutture rauco.

VII. DE UVA GUTTURIS.

Uva madens cum forte modum non continet ipsum,
Extillatque graves putridasque in corpore guttas,
Pulmonisque leves terebrat male sordida pennas,
Siccatur simili citius de pulvere grassans.

VIII. DE PULMONE CURANDO.

Saepe vigens hominis quatitur vis ipsa thoracis,
Cernitur et diram multis intendere mortem.
Si cupis ergo aegrum curis repolire thoracem,
Non pigeat varias herbarum cernere curas.
Lana madens oleo, nec non succus feni Graeci,
Haec reparant stomachum, datus potusque myricae,

Bettonicae celebri sociatur brassica grandis,
Raphanus ex mulsa, dandus prasii quoque succus.
Sumitur et celebris digne lelisphagus herba,
Ultima sic dabitur magnae curatio cedri.

IX. DE CORDIS DOLORE.

Cum dolor insanus lateri praecordia pulsat,
Et cordis fibras multum dolor angit acerbus,
Dira fluenta juvant juncta virtute coralli.
Dein pipinella levis sociatur jure marathri.
Sizaduar capitur, nec non tanaceta virilis,
Quae et sedat febres cordisque venena repulsat.

X. DE PLEURESEOS CURA.

At si forte pium latus pulsaverit ingens
Morbus, et ancipiti turbatur vita periclo,
Accelerare lupi pellem studeas, et ponere caldam,
Cervi et medullam poteris cum unguine capri.
Protinus in cacabo mittantur, igneque lento,
Pix pariter britia societur decoquaturque,
Farris et ipsa lupina simul, et non sine croco.
Sicque malagma pium morbo jungatur acerbo,
Quo requies detur misero nimium laboranti.
Et vitium pellit celebris medicina Tonantis.

XI. DE SPLENIS CURA.

Splen tumidus hominem plaustum cum forte molestat,
Bettonicam coquis, et socias purgata columbae,
Quae duo juncta simul poscunt jungi cephalotam,
Rosaceumque oleum; certus sic madida nectis.
Thymbra brevis rapitur, sociantur atque lupini,
Saepius et dantur, bibitur quoque lingnula cervi,
Qua virtute perit facies, sed blanda rugatur.

Nascitur in petris humilis, sed magna lieni
Est et amica homini, verum haud risibus apta.
Quot sunt membra hominis, tot sunt in corpore pestes.
Sed medicina potens compescit munere multas.
Dum vitiatur hepar gliscitque ex more scyrosis,
Costus acer bibitur, necnon reubarbarus ingens.
Quae contrita simul reprimunt cum sale tumentem.
Fibra lupina valet, juvat ac potata dolenti,
Cum patitur jecur in dextra, splen ipsa sinistra.
Cura ideo amborum parilis conjuncta duobus.

XII. DE STOMACHI ET INTESTINI DOLORIBUS.

Viscera multimodis quatiuntur intima poenis,
Et cruciatur eger totus languore minaci,
Nec spes ulla manet vitae, cum spiritus ipse
Alta petit, peregrinus abit, bona quaeque relinquit.
Dicitur haec torta, gravis quia viscera torquet,
Atque iterum iterumque placat, corrumpitur omnis
Chara natura simul, reparat quod fervida lympha.
Sic pigra ex ipso foveantur membra liquore
Et frigida ex calidis amnentur cuncta fluentis.
Postea distractus fundatur anseris adeps,
Et sociata simul pateat virtus feni Graeci.
Nec minus in liquidis coquitur vis ipsa fluentis.
Protinus et pavidum fundatur clyster in anum,
Qua virtute miser poterit reparare dolorem
Squibala quem faciunt dum non sit cura salubris,
Claudit et angustos patientis cholera cursus.
Raditur et niveus elephas, statim bibiturque,
Distorquet tortos citius haec datio potus.
Sumuntur catuli ut fertur pia viscera caeci,
Mollia sic teneris adhibendum membrula fibris.
Et dolor omnis habrae transitque in viscera fissi.

Plinius id memorat, scimus quem vera locutum.

XIII. DE HYDROPIS CURA.

Ex scyrosi splenis mortalis nascitur humor,
Et segregat miseram misero de viscere pellem,
Tantaque vis morbi est, sitiens ut non satietur.
Sumuntur cineres quos urit fraxinus alta,
Ex his lisciva franguntur hordea dura,
Bis simul excoctis fidus compone dolenti,
Raphanus ex dulci mandatur optima melle,
Cujus ex foliis epithema apponitur ipsum.
Sulphura cum veteri potantur fervida vino:
Nec minus ex ipsis epithema appone tumenti.
Haec scyrosin splenis solvunt, lymphas quoque siccant.

XIV. DE TINEIS.

Putrida sanguineis gliscunt si vulnera morbis,
Conveniet calidum lacte potare caprinum
Nec minus ex asina solvunt apostema dirum.
Vitis amineae cineres funduntur olivo:
Potus hic est putridis multis per saecula dignus.
Ast apium caricaeque simul, nec non baca lauri,
Iris, et Illyrica grandis centauria ruta,
Haec poterunt citius purulentas tergere sordes,
Ac redivivum hominem laetis reparare diebus.

XV. DE VERME AURIS.

Convenit incautis cautas praetendere curas,
Ne minus indocili turbentur corpora sensu.
Cum sopor immensus hominis pervaserit artus,
Tum solet indignas animal penetrarier aures.
Accipe cum cepa citius vel muris aceto,
Nec moram facias, poteris sic pellere vermem.

XVI. DE SURDITATE.

At si surditiam pateris, rubros lege vermes
Arboris antiquae, puro sic miscis olivo;
Auribus infundis, cupidam tibi redde salutem.
Anserinus adeps prodest et vulturis atri.
Ceparum succus juvat auribus et bona praestat,
Cum solet incautis aures pervadere lympha.

XVII. DE DYSENTERIA.

Saepe solet ventris nimius transcurrere cursus,
Paulatim teneram multorum solvere carnem,
Quem prudens medicina Dei compescere noscit.
Galla asiana juvat, cerasi longum quoque pomum,
Caseus aptus erit dulci cum munere mellis,
Proderit et calidum hirci de viscere ruptum
Appositum ventri sevum, quae cognita cura est.
At proprium si forte unguem demittit ab ipso,
Significat citius cupitam jam perdere vitam.

XVIII. DE DURITIA VENTRIS.

Si vero immenso turbatur pondere venter,
Aspice quo crescit venando germine pallas;
Dicitur haec virgo cunctis et amica salutis;
Protinus et capito, gliscit bona gratia ventri.
Elleborum capitur, teritur, mulsum bibiturque,
Semper ad hunc valuit morbum nec non chamaeactis
Diluta cum veteri statim potanda lyaeo.
Proderit et gustus sine mora lactis equini.
Eupator, prasion, atque hermodactylus ipsa,
Fertur ut in libris, semper sunt ventris amici.

XIX. DE VESICA.

Multis multa juvant quia sunt contraria morbis
Morbus ab antidoto superatur numinis alti.
Est morbi species multis inimicaque pestis,
Cum furit insanus vesicae calculus ardens,
Saxa quidem generans quibus cunctatur urina.
Nec valet homo dolens imbres laxare benignos.
Hedera celsa dabit celso de culmine baccas,
Ipsius et succum cum vino sume tepenti,
Nec mora, rumpetur plantago glandis, et ipsa
Sumitur et bibitur olusatrumque benigna.
Saxifricam tollunt petro necnonque selino.
Suffragiis his fultus eris. Dominumque rogabis.

XX. DE FLUXU URINAE.

Quod si contra fluens nimios perfuderit imbres,
Ex cerebro leporis statim compesce fluentem.
Vina vetusta capis, cerebrum cum percipis ipsum,
Vile quidem est potu, sed non medicamine vile.

XXI. DE SANGUINE NARIUM.

Dicendum cunctis cum fundit sanguinis unda
Naris haemorrhoida, quae sit spes certa salutis.
Ruta dabit potum pariter contrita nidorem,
Humilis ex campis prodest contrita cumino
Hypporis, et sistit conjuncta nare cruorem
Pulvere boleti quem fantur esse lupinum,
Naribus associas vilis quoque gramina mentae.

XXI. DE HAEMORRHOIDE.

Si vero obscenum morbus tentaverit anum,
Quaeratur maurella potens inimicaque talpae,
Nec non hyosciamus, quarum fit cura salubris
Haec epota simul sistunt jam jamque cruorem

Plumbus et ustus obest madido conjunctus olivo.
His junctim binis subsistit sanguinis unda.

XXIII. DE IGNE.

Perfurit ignis acer comburens viscera semper,
Semper et errat atrox flammam sub cute remittens
Atque iterum exsiliens fontis sub imagine gliscens.
Fraudibus internis ejus sit obvia semper
Mens hominis; linire juvat chelidoniae gramen.
Internus nivei sociatur candidus ovi,
Ruta juvat morbumque fugat, stringit quoque flammam,
Si tepido puroque simul jungatur olivo.
Ne putes haec quod falsa loquar, cum dicere verum
Veritas ipsa jubet; stercus producito morbo
Ovis et id calidum, referunt quod carmine plures.

XXIV. DE CARBONE.

Vis inimica viget morbus cum perfurit ingens,
Languida terrificus perimit cum viscera carbo.
Jovis huic barbae succus pariterque benignae,
Quae simul est hostis, nec non contrita savina
Stercore cum nitidae potantur jura columbae;
Sumpta quae si tremulo remanent in corporis alvo,
Vita salus pavido sic jam promittitur aegro.
Sin vero exhaustum videtur reicere potum,
Crede mihi celerem videtur pandere mortem.
Hunc etiam dirum raparum semine pelli
Asseruit Quintus vera ratione Serenus.
Prosunt et impressa gravi cauteria morbo,
Calx etiam viva statim conspargitur in quo.
Cumque Dei jussu fuerit rubicunda cicatrix,
Tunc vero intrepidus timidam componito curam,
Quo virulenta lues valeat haurire venena.

Hoc tamen attestor, noscas vitare soporem,
Ne redivivus atrox possit reparare vigorem.

XXV. DE SCIA ARTHRITICA.

Si cui coxendix gressum fraudaverit ipsum,
Ossaque perlustrans furibundus creverit humor,
Sume polypodium quam dicunt esse filiclam,
Cui bene miscetur tritus cariophylus ater
Ductilis et piper, gratum cunctis cynamomum.
Sic potum facias; tribuas sed non sine melle.
Arboris ulmineae discas perquirere librum,
Cui rubiam misceto, simul potato jucundus.
Urticam cernens ruris, ne sperne majorem,
Quae potata diu noscit comburere pestem.
Id teneas certum firmum verum quoque, nate.

XXVI. DE PODAGRA CURANDA.

Multi multa ferunt, quorum scriptura salubris,
Qui tamen affirmant pigram sine cura podagram,
Dicere si potis est; si vis succurrere morbo,
Incipe quod moneo; gratos succidito lactes.
Sic dolor immanis novit superare dolorem.
Felicis appositum requiem dat gressibus unguen
Et myrica potens, vivens quoque barbula Jovis,
Pinsuntur pariter, pedibus nectuntur, et ipsae
Carpuntur jugiter claudo potum tribuentes.
Vis tibi mirificam jam nunc mandare salutem?
Pisciculos capito spinae ruccas nomine dictos.
Quos lateri impositos ferventibus addito prunis,
Gressibus ac certus calidos compone dolentis;
Omne malum reprimunt, pestis sic dura fugatur.

CRISPI MEDIOLANENSIS DIACONI AD MACRUM MANTUENSEM PRAEPOSITUM EXPLICIT. SED PROFECTO CRISPUS ISTE NEQUE POETA EST NEC VERSIFICATOR BONUS; QUIPPE NON EX LEGE METRORUM SED AD SUARUM AURIUM SONUM VERSUS COMPOSUIT, ID EST RHYTHMUM TANTUM.

ΤΕΛΟΣ.

This work was produced in association with:

THE SCRIPTORIUM PROJECT

DALCASSIAN PRESS

Dark Age & Medieval Texts

Wilmington, DE

www.ingramcontent.com/pod-product-compliance
Lightning Source LLC
LaVergne TN
LVHW050940210926
848482LV00013B/683